FA[illegible]

MANY PEOPLE who s[illegible] depression are rather ashamed of it. They think that they ought to be able to pull themselves out of it by prayer and willpower, and when their efforts just make things worse they get still more depressed and more ashamed. Many others do not even realise what is wrong with them. I have made it a habit to ask those who come to see me about difficulties with prayer and similar problems a few question about their feelings, their sleep pattern and so on, and in a great many cases it becomes obvious that the real problem is depression, even though they have not thought of it in these terms. It can be a tremendous relief to such people to have their feelings brought out into the open, recognised and talked about, and to discuss positive ways of coping with them.

So it seems worthwhile to try to put on paper my own experience of depression and the ways in which I myself try to cope with it and pray in it, in the hope that it will help both those who have this illness themselves and those who find themselves trying to counsel or direct people who are suffering from it. It is, I know, immensely difficult for those who naturally have a cheerful, sanguine sort of temperament to enter into a depressed person's experience and stand with them in it. Even psychiatrists seldom seem really to understand what it feels like, so a first-hand account may help. Inevitably, the account is written when the experience itself has lightened a little and has become recent memory rather than present fact, so it is difficult to be certain that I am not exaggerating or understating my feelings; but I have done my best to be honest.

I

I get very fed up with doctors who ask me what I am depressed about because it is my experience that a person in depression is not depressed *about* anything. He is just depressed, and it is extremely difficult to describe what that means. Sometimes, when the depression is fairly acute, everything does seem black, gloomy and certainly hopeless. For myself, there is always the temptation to contract out or to retire; sometimes to contract out of engagements to which I am committed, and sometimes just to retire and be alone—certainly often to retire from my job, which does not seem worth going on with. I feel that the best thing for everyone would be if I got out altogether, and therefore I even think vaguely of suicide, which would be the ultimate contracting out. But most of the time it is not as bad as that. It is possible to put a good face on everyday life, but everything seems an octave, or two or three octaves, too low. I simply cannot try hard enough and any effort to do so ends in failure and therefore in more depression.

In some ways the most physically obvious sign of depression is real tiredness, weariness of mind and body, and this of course even affects my walk so that I tend to slouch and drag my feet even more than I normally do. Perhaps the most acute mental sign is an utter loneliness and desolation which I am not able to describe. A lot of this is self-inflicted, because I have friends and could seek companionship, but somehow when I am in this state I prefer to be alone and indulge in the isolation and desolation. With this there goes an absolutely unreasoning, angry aggression, particularly to those close to me and whom I love. This ties up with what those psychiatrists say who maintain that all depression is repressed rage. Certainly I cannot really separate them in my own mind.

Another aspect of this is that I get hypersensitive towards any criticism, no matter how slight, and this is accompanied by self-justification—always to myself and sometimes expressed—so that I keep on seeking for approval and praise, and particularly for 'success' in terms of numbers in church, and so on. Any obvious failure very much deepens my depression and anger, as does any form of rejection. When I give advice to people in the smallest things—that a particular book might help them, for instance, and in fact it fails to do so—I get angry and hurt that my suggestion has not been acceptable. I know with my intellect that this is completely stupid, but that is no help because the source of depression lurks not in the intellect but in the guts, along with fear and anger and hate. Of course, the opposite is true as well. Not only am I hypersensitive to failure and rejection, but I myself reject any advice and help which is offered to me (though I do at least have the sense to see a psychiatrist regularly and take the medicine he prescribes).

Another very unpleasant aspect of depression is that although it is an illness and has its origin in the subconscious mind—in the guts—it also rubs one's nose in actual and real guilt for sins and failures. It has forced me to face the conscious guilt of my consistent sin and sins and sinfulness and my refusal to stop sinning: my refusal to sacrifice things I know I ought to sacrifice. These are at very many levels from the grossly physical to the more subtle selfishnesses. In my depression I have found out some very horrible things about myself—and that is not being pseudo-humble or more of a hypocrite than I can help. I know exactly, for instance, what 'hardness of heart' means and it is a very terrifying thing indeed.

II

As I have said, when I am seriously depressed, I think vaguely about suicide. I do not think that I have seriously considered it since I became a Christian, although I certainly did on at least two occasions before that. But the idea of suicide does come into my mind, as it inevitably will in a real depression. On these occasions it is useful to have worked out in your mind some solid reasons why you should not commit suicide. Even though they may not mean much then, you know that they did mean something once, and will again, and you have something to hang on to. It is also useful to have these points in mind when talking to severely depressed people. Obviously they cannot be trotted out in a neat logical row, but sometimes one or another will make sense to the person you are talking to.

One reason, which would probably be more valid to a person who has some kind of belief in God, is that my life is not my own. Suicide is often thought of as 'taking my own life', but my own life is something which I have not got. I did not 'get' my life. It was given to me. I may or may not believe it was given to me by God, but in any case I got it from my parents, and someone took quite a lot of trouble to make sure that I survived and grew up. I am part of a form of existence, part of the human race, and I am a unique part. No one else is like me and no one else can stand in for me. Further, if I believe in God and commit suicide I am really saying, 'Look, God, you made a mistake and there is nothing you can do about it. The thing is such a mess that it is beyond all hope. I cannot bear it and you cannot help me'. In other words, suicide is the ultimate blasphemy. In terms of this life, at least, it puts beyond possibility the turning and accepting forgiveness—that forgiveness we call repentance. It cannot put us beyond God's infinite love (and I believe most suicides are so agonised that they are especially deeply loved by God) but killing myself does destroy the possibility of receiving that forgiveness in this life—suicide puts me 'beyond' repentance.

Suicide is also a completely selfish act, the act of what the Greeks call *idios*, which means a person completely private and alone (whence our word idiot). It rejects all those who need me, who love me, who have tried to help me—and most depressed people do not realise how numerous these may be. (I still remember with pain and guilt, after nearly forty years, a man who shot himself after he had come to me for help). It is *never* true to say, 'they are better off without me', even though there may be some financial or physical benefit in my death.

That is the negative side. On the positive side, it helps to hang on to even one thing which makes life worth living, something which I can still enjoy, or have enjoyed and may be able to again—whether it is music or sunrise or sunset, or a friend's company or a drink. It is also a help, if you are talking to someone who is depressed, to try to help them to see and believe that there is something about them which is really likeable—worth having in the world—whether it is a gift for friendship, or quietness, or a nice smile, or an attractive shape—something which they themselves can admit, however reluctantly, 'Yes, that is something I have got or can do'—it does not really matter what. Finally, it is worth remembering, when you feel right down at the very, very bottom, that at least it is somewhere from which you can start again. Nothing can get worse, so it might get at least a bit better.

III

The first thing to do when you become depressed is to accept the fact. It really is no good struggling against it, and the very worst thing to do from every point of view, physical, psychological and spiritual, is to be depressed about being depressed, or resentful about it or angry about it (easier said than done, I know).

Having accepted the fact that you are depressed, the next thing is to go to a doctor, if possible a psychiatrist. (I heard a GP say on a TV programme about depression in which I took part some time ago, that he had been a GP for twenty-five years and really knew nothing about depression at all). You simply ought not to mess about with depression since it can be a very serious illness indeed, and have all sorts of side-effects on your physical health, your job and those who are close to you. I agree that there is no point in living on pills but it is stupid not to use them when they are needed and there are very good anti-depressants available which have enabled me to live with these depressions for a number of years—so use them if they are prescribed. Some people think it wrong to take medicine, especially for states which do not appear to have a physical cause, on the grounds that 'the grace of God should be sufficient'. Certainly the grace of God is all-sufficient, but we do not know at any given moment in our lives how or by what means the grace of God will operate, and it may well be that medicine or skilled treatment—which are not opposed to grace—can provide channels for grace when we humbly admit our need of the help they can give. For little as we know about depression, it is known that some types have a physical cause, or can at least be physically alleviated, while others may have a psychological cause which can be got at and dealt with by trained people.

Neither is it helpful to say that Christians ought not to be depressed. Perhaps it is true we ought not to be, but it is no good telling us not to be what we are! And so another piece of practical advice is not to try and cheer up, no matter what your well-meaning friends may say. Cheerful books and magazines, light-hearted parties and so on seem to make things worse, not better. Instead, I find it a help to read and listen to things which echo the way I am feeling and are in tune with it—deep music, like that so often written for the cello, poems by writers who know themselves what depression feels like. (Parts of Coleridge's 'Ancient Mariner' are very good for this but there is much else besides.) For some reason this verse by Roy Batt 'fits' exactly for me:

> A broken heart does best
> In a well-appointed room
> With knick-knacks here and there
> And a discreet rose in bloom.
> Calamities of heart and sense
> Befit pretence.

The right kind of picture can also help. I find it comforting to look at dark Rembrandts with their sad, experienced faces and heavy shadows; and to repeat the words of David on the death of his son, 'Oh, my son Absalom, my son, my son Absalom! ... my son, my son!' It is partly the cadence which echoes the low rhythm of depression and partly that this is the cry of a man in agony. And without trying to be dramatic, depression is an agony and it makes it less lonely to know that others have shared the pain.

IV

For those who are Christians, or who are at least prepared to call out, however angrily, to God or fate in their pain, depression affords an opportunity of discovering 'God in the guts' which might not otherwise occur. Both Old and New Testaments have quite a lot to say about basic emotions which are below conscious control, using words like 'bowels' and 'reins' (which generally means kidneys). In I Maccabees 2, when the father was asked to sacrifice to an idol he said his 'reins trembled', and the Psalmist says, 'My heart was grieved. It went even through my reins, so foolish was I and ignorant, even as a beast before thee' (Ps. 73:20). And in the Authorised Version of the New Testament, the Epistles several times use the word 'bowels' for feelings too deep for words. On the other hand, the AV often uses 'heart' to represent the more conscious, more articulate part of feelings, the *ego* rather than the *id*, perhaps. We are told to lift up our hearts, whereas it is inconceivable that we should lift up our guts. But the point is that when we are down there in the depths, unable to lift ourselves or to be lifted, He stays down there with us in the depression—He abides in us and we in Him, even down there. Indeed, in some way it is easier to find God in the depths than in the heights. 'If I climb up into heaven, thou art there' is all very well but it does mean climbing, it means discipline and hard work and sacrifice. But 'if I go down into hell, thou art there also.' It does not need any effort to go down, and in the sort of hell depression is, He is certainly there. He does not seem to give any comfort and strength that one can feel consciously, but there is somehow a closeness to reality, which brings one closer to basic fact of things, to God who is the basic fact of all being and all existence.

An analogy which helps me personally in thinking about this is the neutron star. This is the kind of star which burns itself out by throwing off its protons and everything else and thus becomes total emptiness, what is called, 'infinite gravity', the dead centre, the total stillness at the heart of the whirlpool which yet sucks in everything around it. This, it seems to me, is the epitome of depression and in some ways also a picture of the meaning of the cross. It is to that still centre that depression can bring us. Or, to take another analogy, it feels like being buried deep in the soil where there is no sunlight, or smothered in heavy, wet, dark jungle. These are places where things grow, however dark or dangerous they may be. So, although I can hardly welcome being depressed, I keep on hoping that the next time it happens, I will be able to deal with it a bit more positively than I did the last time, and that I shall be able to gain something from it and grow in it.

V

It will be clear from what I have just written that I believe it is essential to keep praying in depression, not just hanging on to the lifeline of my normal rule of prayer, vital though that is, but also, as and how I can, using my tiredness and anger and despair to realise my total dependence on God. When I feel utterly useless and worthless and unable of my own will to do anything at all, I really know from experience—and not just with my intellect—that I do not have any existence except through the continual maintaining and sustaining power of God's love. I am ensconced in God, encapsulated, encradled in His love (that is what that great poem, 'St Patrick's Breastplate' is about). His love penetrates through every fibre of every being—spirit, soul and body—and so all created things, including my empty self, reflect the glory of that love. It may be a dark glory, not glamorous or gorgeous, but it is there within me. I am held in being, sustained and covered by Him.

So, in the hopelessness and meaninglessness and depression, when the guiding beacon of God's glorious transcendence vanishes, it is possible to glimpse the immanence of God 'inside' and to discover that the search for meaning, the search for oneself and the search for God are finally all the same thing. It is in the depths that 'our lives are hid with Christ in God'.

In that seeking inwards to the centre of being, the words of the Psalms can be a great support:

> 'O knit my heart unto thee, that I may fear thy name.'
>
> (87:11.)

> 'For innumerable troubles are come about me; my sins have taken such hold upon me that I am not able to look up: yea, they are more in number than the hairs of my head, and my heart hath failed me.' (40:15.)

> 'I stretch forth my hands unto thee: my soul gaspeth unto thee as a thirsty land.' (143:6.)

> 'The Lord himself is the portion of mine inheritance and my lot.' (16:6.)

> 'He made darkness his secret place: his pavilion round about him, with dark waters and thick clouds to cover him.' (18:11.)

> 'He shall send down from on high to fetch me: and shall take me out of many waters.' (18:16.)

Countless passages from the Psalms could be quoted, especially all of Psalms 27 and 42, as well as much of Isaiah; while many other parts of both Old and New Testaments are, it need hardly be said, wonderfully strengthening in depression. But what speaks to one person will not speak to another and you have to search for yourself.

Conclusion

So I come full circle to what, as I have already said, is for me the basic urge in depression—the urge to run away, to retreat, to get out. But ultimately you cannot run from yourself, except by suicide (and even that is uncertain since we do not know what happens after that), and so the only way to go is inwards and downwards, to the depths of one's own being. And if that is where you retreat to, He is there. For those who 'going through the vale of misery use it for a well' the pools are filled with water, and not only with water but with pearls of great price and buried treasure. And although I would not wish the agony of depression on anyone, those of us who suffer from it can, if we are willing to, find depths which seem in some ways to be comparable to the heights which the mystics reach.

Of course, part of the trouble is that if you found these riches while you were depressed you would not be depressed. It is only when you are through the worst (at least for a time) that you realise what it has meant. In the same way, I could not have written this essay when things were really bad. But I hope it may be a help to those who are struggling with this particular kind of torment, or are trying to help others to do so.

Also by Gonville ffrench-Beytagh

OUT OF THE DEPTHS

Encountering Depression

> *Experiences of darkness, depression, dereliction are so much a part of maturing into the depths of friendship with God. We need people who can be true to their experience and share it with us.*
>
> 'Epilogue', Wendy Robinson

Since its first publication in 1990, this candid, personal account of depression, and recovery from 'out of the depths', has helped many to come to terms with their own experiences, or provide support to other sufferers. It was by continuing to say the Psalms and read the Bible, through force of habit, that the author discovered voices which penetrated his darkness and confusion.

Wendy Robinson, the writer of the Epilogue, pays a warm tribute to Gonville ffench-Beytagh, with whom she shares an understanding of the challenge presented by depression for the Church and for the Christian faith. As a Christian and a psychotherapist, she contributes her own insights into the nature and treatment of depression, and its liberating potential.

Fairacres Publications 162 ISBN 978-0-7283-0183-2
Price: £4.00 ISSN 0307-1405